A Fine Summer in Chicago

Table of Contents

A Fine Summer in Chicago

Preface

Chicago is a life-changing city. Last year in 2015, my classmates and I began medical school at one of the most prestigious universities in the world. That said, here are a few things you should know:

I am African American.
This is not a story about violence.
This is a work of non-fiction. Many of the names in this story, including my own, have been changed.

The events that I will recount took place during the summer of 2016. As happens annually, the majority of the class stayed on after our first year to work on research projects with mentors of our choosing. I chose to work in an ovarian cancer research lab. My aim was to determine whether mesothelial cells treated with an optimal dose of Compound X, an antioxidant found in the skins of various fruits and vegetables, have reduced affinity to ovarian cancer cells.

My name is Dil Lewis. Just to let you know, these are the people that won recognition for their work at the end of the summer:

Emeka Woods
Leo Lawson
Dianna Flowers
Joann Chin
Teresa Wade
William Alexander
Pete White
Doyle Mcgee
Felicia Ramirez

A Fine Summer in Chicago

Mamie Green
Patricia Frazier
Greg Norris
Ronnie Black
Claire Johnston
Marcus Rios
Ruben Harrison
Nick Lindsey
Charlene Garcia

Like the majority of my classmates, I was not recognized for my summer work with an award. Yet, why do I feel that I gained so much?

This story is about the summer that changed my life.

A Fine Summer in Chicago

The Spring

"Nice to meet you." Colin Law, chairman of Obstetrics and Gynecology, responded. We were beginning a conversation about working in his ovarian cancer research lab during the summer. He sat, hands folded and both feet planted, carrying the dignified air of a physician with a global reputation. Colin is an Italian physician, having received both his MD and PhD in Germany. It's fair to say that he is one of the smartest guys, if not the smartest, in any room he happens to find himself. Dr. Law had given us a talk during the pelvic section of our anatomy course late in the previous summer, outlining the surgical aspects of his daily work as a gynecologic oncologist. With respect and barely contained composure, I listened as my future mentor described the radical vaginal trachelectomy, a surgical technique that excises the cervix but preserves the uterus, enabling cervical cancer patients of child-bearing age to deliver healthy children. "Performing these surgeries is one of the most satisfying things I've been able to do in my life," he had added. Looking around the room that September, I was sold. I didn't know what was keeping people in their chairs.

"So, have you all taken biochemistry?" Colin asked in our meeting that April. I had taken the course that fall. When I told him so, he then inquired, "and do they have grades for those courses or is it pass/no pass?" Many medical schools across the country have transitioned to a pass/fail pre-clinical curriculum. In my opinion, it facilitates a work-life balance, as well as a more collaborative environment. I described this to him. He shifted uneasily. I could have told him my absolute scores for the exams in the biochemistry course, but I decided to hold my peace. Colin then went on to mention that he had received interest from two other students in joining his lab for the summer. "But, we didn't give away your spot." Admittedly, it was a bit surprising that my email to him and Grace Ramsey (my primary mentor for day to day lab

A Fine Summer in Chicago

guidance) that February had sealed my entrance to the lab as the first student to show interest. This is because medical students tend to be an anxiously driven breed. "Early and often" is the motto by which many of us live. I'd been interested in working with Colin since that fateful day in September, after his compelling lecture. In fact, I'd even began sitting in on a few lab meetings in October and November, taking in the environment. Still, when he said those words to me, I felt a deep sense of gratitude. At least one of the other two students expressing interest, I would later find out, had research experiences that far eclipsed my own cell culturing experiences. Giving them preference would have been very understandable.

"Thank you sir." My immediate response. "Grace will be your primary contact. Let me know..." To be honest, I don't recall the rest of the conversation. A flood of thoughts flashed before me. Memories of ambitious researchers from my past rejecting my request to join their basic science labs. Back then, I lacked both research experience as well as the fundamental coursework to understand what I would be researching. Yet, here now was this well-established researcher taking me on. What had changed? First, I was now a medical trainee. Now that I was studying medicine, I was going to become a member of a privileged group within Western society. It is a membership that comes with benefits that, through a built-in summer research session, I was already beginning to realize. Second, I now expressed interest in simply learning. Even if I did not develop the cure for ovarian cancer during the upcoming summer, I hoped to get the most out of my experience. One last reason that I think the winds of change had blown in my favor was that I was now in Chicago, a city that has given birth to and nurtured many inspiring and diverse leaders, many of whom seek to inspire and diversify the fields in which they have been so fortunate to succeed. It was with these truths in mind, and with a sense of gratitude, that I marched ahead that spring to develop the skills to succeed in research.

A Fine Summer in Chicago

Inauspicious Beginnings

Science is incredible. But it has only one problem. It requires human beings to perform. Take the Bicinchoninic Acid (BCA) assay, for example. Fixed volumes of various concentrations of different protein standards of known concentration, protein samples of unknown concentration, and proteins are added to wells in a culture plate in order to calculate the equation of a standard line used to determine how much protein should be added to a lane for a Western Blot (WB). Learning this technique is the foundation for quantifying how much of a specific protein is available in a cell.

We perform the BCA with the understanding that there will be variability in the amount of protein pipetted between different wells. A regression statistic, or R^2 value, examines this variability. This value ranges from 0 to 1. So R^2 value of 0 indicates absolute variability, while R^2 value of 1 indicates no variability. Generally, we want this value to be 0.97 or higher when calculating protein concentrations for our WB. The trouble is that variability exists in pipetting *everything*. As Tim Peterson, a post-doctoral (post-doc) scholar in our lab, puts it--"even if you're perfect, the pipet isn't." Once you've loaded the protein with the proper reagents, researchers usually give 30 minutes to an hour to let the protein react with the reagents, forming a purple hue. We then quantify the amount of reacted protein with a spectrophotometer. The darker the hue of purple, the more protein is present.

In the spring of 2016, I learned this, alongside many other techniques that I won't delve into now, in preparation for the summer, from Spencer Graham.

Spencer Graham is a research technician who had worked in the Law Lab for 2 and a half years. He had graduated in 2013, the same year as I, from the University of Rochester with a degree in

A Fine Summer in Chicago

Biology. Spencer and I were the same age, and had hit it off pretty quickly. He is about 5'9", Caucasian, and had run track for a couple years in college. My go-to guy for experimental questions during the spring and summer, he instructed me on how to perform the BCA assay. In his lessons, he would say with a smile, "First, you have to hold a pipet like this. Not the way you like to hold it." We would both laugh. Of course, when I mentioned I had a dearth of experience, you now understand that I hadn't learned how to properly hold a micro-pipet before. In fact, when first learning that spring, I realized I'd been holding it backwards.

I think that everyone should work in a research lab before they turn 25 years old. This is true for three main reasons:

1. We need more scientists. More minds=More breakthroughs.
2. I believe we should understand what we dislike just as much as what we enjoy. Even if one is put off by the idea of pipetting, culturing cells, or handling various chemicals in the hopes of advancing scientific inquiry, how can one know for sure unless they actually sit down and do an experiment?
3. Science is frustrating. I performed over 100 experiments last summer. How many did I present? 10. "We publish 2 to 3% of all experiments we perform in this lab," Colin says. The frustration builds an element of resilience when things go wrong, but exhilaration when experiments return positive results. A spiritual perspective: Ecclesiastes 7:14-When times are good, be happy; but when times are bad, consider this: God has made the one as well as the other. Therefore, no one can discover anything about their future.

Spencer did well on the MCAT, and was preparing applications to medical school. He had a deep understanding of concepts unrelated to medicine. He knew a ton about photography, the benefits of varying exposure lengths, and could describe the nuances of how lighting impacted the quality of a photograph. He

A Fine Summer in Chicago

knew details about bikes, soccer, running...and the list goes on. Plus, he was a nice guy and willing to teach others—in short, the perfect classmate. It was a privilege to work with Spencer. Working with him helped me develop a capacity for teaching, which of course comes in handy when educating patients. However, I am glad that medical schools are selecting for individuals like him, and go further to refine the qualities he had: skills in the sciences, but also a working knowledge of the humanities, athletics, and most importantly, themselves.

It was this self- knowledge that sticks out to me the most. He knew what he cared about, what things were vital to him. Assessing myself, I knew that it was imperative to give the project my best effort. How could I not? Especially, in light of what Colin did for me, accepting me into the lab. Working hard in the face of challenge is easier said than done, of course. As the spring progressed, the crucible of research life rocked my world. I would watch helplessly as dyed proteins glide into the incorrect lane, or I saw 2 days of WB procedure culminate in unreadable schmutz.

During those times, I was reminded of a scene from Denzel Washington's film, *Remember the Titans*. Coach Boone, the new African American high school football coach, walks into a crowded gymnasium of black football players. Pete, a talented running back, has his hand raised to give his new black head coach a high-five before their meeting. Coach Boone looks at him with his stern stare, and ultimately makes a fool of young Pete, asking him why he is smiling, why he thinks football is fun. You see, I was Pete. Our Lab was my gymnasium. The pipet was my Coach Boone.

Once I realized that working in the lab was going to be a challenge, I talked with Tim about the upcoming challenges. "You get out what you put in, right?" I remember asking. "It's true," he says. "We only make this look easy because we have been around and messed up enough times." I took a tiny bit of comfort in that.

A Fine Summer in Chicago

Fits and Starts

The seas of the summer started off smooth enough. It was at this time that I began to get acclimated to being in the lab full time. The primary task was to build knowledge of the literature during that first week. My initial goal from the spring had been to study and characterize levels of Protein Y in relation to other proteins in the cell. I was more than happy to begin doing so. Grace, the junior PI in her mid-30s to whom I looked for guidance, was looking out for me all the time. There was quite a bit of literature to suggest that there might not be significant new findings contributing to the literature. Based on feedback from the administration responsible for approving my summer research, the project was "too ambitious." It might have been a bit challenging, or at least challenging for a guy who didn't even know how to hold a micropipette, to produce significant findings after just 10 weeks. You can begin to see why I appreciate the confidence that Colin, my senior PI put in me then. "I don't lower my standards for anybody," he notes.

In any case, a secondary aim looking at Compound X, the antioxidant of interest, was proposed for study after the first 2 weeks of summer. To assess its efficacy, I modified the project to measure the activity of Protein Y, up-regulated due to oxidative stress. It's actually more exciting than it sounds. That being said, in order to feel relevant to ovarian cancer, a condition diagnosed after metastasis in over 70 percent of cases, I needed to make sure that I was looking at process associated with ovarian cancer metastasis. These include: the ability of the ovarian cancer cells to adhere, invade, and proliferate on the mesothelial cell layer. It's here that I should introduce my independent study group leaders. Frank Chuahan, MD,PhD; Elisia Boateng, MD; and Alexis Truong, PhD. Elisia and Alexis tended to speak in paragraphs, while Frank was a bit more reserved, focusing more on important high points. Yet all were very pleasant, attentive, and gentle in their guidance. Alexis and Frank were the individuals that mentioned that they were more inspired by my secondary aim, and that I should instead make it my primary focus (instead of studying Protein Y). Research is quite circuitous, but we have to be flexible.

To keep a balance, I made sure to keep up with my friends periodically over dinner. Naturally, we'd commiserate about the amorphous nature of our research projects. I'd later find out that a friend of mine had been drinking a beer each night with the specific purpose of forgetting about the day. He stopped doing so after 2 weeks, citing fear of slipping into dependency. I realized that the emotions we experience in uncertainty are strong. It's necessary as budding physicians to understand this, to embrace the hectic external pressures and circumstances we all face. For example, I co-coordinate a student-led free medical clinic. One of my faculty physician-volunteers has a son that passed away unexpectedly in June. The principal goal of the profession I am studying to join is to preserve life. What happens when we fail our patients? Or they just don't get the chance to be exposed to therapy? Hard questions with which the physician must wrestle. Yet, as a consequence of the spectrum of motivations that God has given us, we desperately arm ourselves with the knowledge we need, and we humble ourselves to learn.

Colin pulled me aside after the first day of the summer for coffee. He wanted to explain the principles by which students that have come into the lab before me, as well as he himself, have been successful. There were three main points:

1. "I turn my phone off and let the world blow up around me."
2. "Stay focused. Shawn Cummings (last year's summer student) was so focused he didn't even know I was around." By the way, Shawn was recognized with an award last year. So was the student that was in our lab before him.

3. "Read one academic paper a day. You have to steal the knowledge here, because we don't pay you enough money. That also means asking everyone in the lab what experiments they are working on, and what their goals are."

High expectations are good for us. It helped set the pace for my summer.

A Fine Summer in Chicago

Nature of the Beauty

Most days over the summer I'd wake up at a decent hour (about 6am) before going through a morning routine. First on the agenda is an incredible devotional by Paul David Tripp, titled *New Morning Mercies.* Each day of the year has its own special message. I found it helpful, gathering grace-directing thoughts to begin the day. Without it I tend to just wander through random scriptures, not actively thinking about applications to my daily life. After scripture time, came my morning workout. Among many other features, the main beauty of the Chicago summers are the placid views of the lake shore superimposed on the early morning sunrise.It is one of the subtle attractions in the windy city. But you have to wake for it. In a city well known for corruption, crime, and segregation, it's nature, that becomes the great equalizer for its citizens. Thankfully, the gorgeous scenery is not limited to the natural environment. Caucasians from the "gold coast", or Northern wealthy portion of the city, often greet African Americans cycling up to the city with a warm smile and wave on their daily runs. I've seen African Americans gladly stop and help visitors seeking directions to a restaurant, or the White Sox game. I am reminded often of Matthew 7:12: "So in everything, do to others what you would have them do to you, for this sums up the Law and the Prophets." Granted, normalizing race relations in Chicago, as I have already alluded, is a fermentation process just past its infancy. Both institutional policy change and personal introspection are important steps we must take to reach that distant promised land. That being said, it is helpful to cite the incremental achievements we make along the way.

The Chicago summers taught me that this introspection should stay with us at all times. A friend of mine, Kate Temple, and I were chatting at a bonfire in mid-June. The fire was dying out, commensurate with the blackening of old newspapers. She and I talked in between bites of smores--mostly about our anticipation of the busyness of summer. She is about my age, though a year ahead in our program. Kate is also a nice, thoughtful, freckled brunette and cares deeply about her faith, her mother(divorced), and her pets. At the time we spoke, she was writing an academic paper that was born out of the research she had done for her summer research project. "I really don't like writing," she says. "It just takes so much time." In short conversations like ours, the prescribed path of least resistance is to simply agree. Instead, I went in the opposite direction. "Well, I do," I respond. "Writing is great. There is so much literature out there on [my topic]. The only way for me to get my head around the mountain of literature is to actually write about it." You can tell we're good friends.

"That's interesting that you say that," Kate says. I think she was a bit stressed about starting her clinical rotations the following Monday. Of course, she did not express as much. I have been impressed with the investment of time she makes, working on developing those ideals which matter most to her. A 2015-2016 Schweitzer fellow (200 hours' community service), it is clear that there was not a ton of time in her days to accomplish all she had on her plate and still have such a robust social life. In fact, my friends and I joke that whenever we see her around that we've witnessed a rare "Kate-sighting."

All joking aside, I sometimes suspect that similar to the way I synthesized my thoughts through writing, distilling the ovarian cancer literature into some form of coherency, Kate believed in "writing" a coherent life narrative by spending time volunteering with her church, seeing her mother often, and playing with her dog—sometimes at the expense of forming stronger friendships, or developing a romantic life. As these thoughts wandered through my consciousness, I notice the sun beginning to set, in all its natural Midwestern glory. Sensing that our conversation, like the sunset, was near, I add a few words. "Well, I would like to do as well as Shawn did, but if I don't get that lucky, then I want to

A Fine Summer in Chicago

work at least as hard as he did last year."

A Fine Summer in Chicago

Late Nights

You should know how the ovarian cancer adhesion, invasion, and proliferation experiments work before I discuss them any further.

I'd first thaw a small tube with a few million mesothelial cells (isolated from our patient's abdominal cavities with full informed consent) into a flask, where I'd usually let them recover for 24-48 hours. I then transferred them to a special plate containing 96 wells. The mesothelial cells are left alone for 24 hours to attach. After 24 hours, a special ovarian cancer cell line is co-plated on top of the mesothelial cell layer for 1-4 hours. I finish up the process by decanting (inverted the plate) any non-adherent cells.[1] Of note, what is special about the cancer cells, is that they were transfected with DNA coding for Green Fluorescence Protein (GFP). That is, DNA isolated from Aequorea Victoria jellyfish. The Nobel Prize-receiving technique was developed by scientists in order to differentiate between labeled and unlabeled cells. Remember the central dogma of biology is that DNA is transcribed to RNA, which is transcribed to Protein. Expression of proteins from the newly transfected DNA enables cells to emit a green fluorescent signal when the cells are exposed to light within specific wavelengths of the electromagnetic spectrum.[2] Over the summer, I learned to quantify the fluorescent cells using a fluorescent cytometer. Science is elegant. However, as I said before, the only problem is that the framework in which it is conducted is imperfect. Cells have variability in their distribution within the container from which they are being drawn, there is error from well to well as the pipet may accumulate bubbles, etc., etc., etc. But the thousands of scientists out there continue to develop new life-saving measures with the mountains of literature accumulating through this process.

Invasion works by co-plating the cells using the processes above, except a special insert is utilized, containing 8 micron pores, that is pre-plated 24 hours prior with a layer of collagen. The ovarian cancer cells are given 24 hours to invade through the mesothelial cells and the collagen layer. The cancer cells on the bottom of the insert can then be fixed and counted either manually or using fluorescent cytometry.[3] Proliferation works similar to adhesion, except that ovarian cancer cells are allowed to grow for 96 hours.[1]

My (now) primary objective for the summer was to determine whether Compound X could reduce or ideally, prevent ovarian cancer adhesion, invasion, or proliferation. The experiment I performed was to treat the mesothelial cells with various doses for various lengths of time to determine whether there were significant differences in the fluorescent cancer cell count in the experimental vs the control group. The lower the number of green cells, the more efficacious the treatment. As you can imagine, this whole process can take up to 1 week at a time, from thaw to reading the proliferation assay. I knew that the summer was going to be a bit hectic, so I threw myself headlong into this project, sometimes culturing 3 to 4 patients at a time. The whole summer, I utilized the recommended doses found in the literature, treating the cells with compound X for 1 week. I tried this for several weeks, but there was no real difference between the experimental and control groups. From an experimental standpoint this was frustrating, so I decided to give the ovarian cancer cells a higher dose of the treatment at the time they were plated. The challenge of course, was how to present data that was growing increasingly complicated.

I was in the cell culture room the evening of August 5th. It was one of those 16-hour days. At about 7:30pm, Grace walks in and exclaims with a hint of hesitation, "I know you don't want to hear this right now, but you will need to redo your results section." "Gosh," I said. "That's a bummer." She wanted to know how long I'd be in the cell culture hood for. I estimated the standard "20 to 30 minutes". Of course, as much as I hope, it never turns out to be

A Fine Summer in Chicago

a 20 to 30-minute job. In fact, the post-docs in the lab and I joked that there was a "time warp" that occurs when I entered the cell culture hood, where 45-minute jobs turned into 12-hour jobs, and that I needed to start paying rent given all the time I'd spent in the hood. I went along with these jokes to make light of the situation, sometimes feeling a sense of guilt for obstructing the work flow of others. Still, I am glad folks were good sports about the learning process. When I found time to meet later to discuss her points of feedback, as it was getting late. Grace spent a large chunk of time with me, walking through the best format to present my data, while bearing with me through any stray comments saturated with naïvetée, even while responsible for other trainees that came and went. Like all things, experiments have a learning curve requiring patience from the experimenter. That being said, Grace was instrumental in helping me gain the confidence I needed through failed experiments. Success would ultimately come, however.

Looking back, I am struck by my luck. I was receiving all of this training, and I was the one getting paid for the experience. The school's arrangement with the NIH allowed us the luxury of a sizable stipend to support our research endeavors. I was fortunate enough to be gainfully learning. No matter how many hours it took to get the job done, I knew I was the lucky one.

A Fine Summer in Chicago

Time Out

As you might have imagined by now. There was not a ton of time in those 16-hour days to see my classmates. Plenty of days would go by without seeing a single medical student. A friend of mine, Sartaj Singh, always kept me in the loop about the goings-on with the medical school community, effectively serving as a social life-line when things got too hectic. Knowing him allowed me to keep a finger on the general medical school pulse, allowing to see students I might not normally see, but with whom I love to interact with on a regular basis. We'd get together in last minute fashion for movies, or Thai food over the weekends, sometimes on 2 hr breaks from the lab. But I still saw him and others when I could.

I'll also tell you about another important experience. There was a small group of 4th grade children at an elementary school in the South Side that a few classmates and I formally mentored through a program known as the South Side Science Scholars(S4). During the year, we taught them about scientific subjects related to everything ranging from the environment to astronomy to biology. It was a deeply satisfying experience. So much so that my buddy coordinating our program, Hank Velasquez, along with his girlfriend (now fiance) Lisette, planned a day trip to the White Sox vs. Tigers baseball game. It was a nice experience. This is mostly because my understanding of baseball was on par with that of the 9 year-old children we were with. It was also interesting because when we arrived, they were already in the 7th inning. Confused, we kept watching. After some time, I overheard a gentleman next to us informing his children about the rain-out the previous night, and how they had to delay the end of the game due to the heavy summer rains. 45 minutes after we arrived, the fireworks went off as a ground ball by the white sox led their players to home base, and to a win. After a brief intermission, snacks, and a bathroom break, the next game began. The Sox won that one as well. It was a good day. But what are the chances?

I also went to Minneapolis over the 4th of July, staying with a friend of mine, Rajat Anu. Rajat was born in India, moving to the United States for his undergraduate education, where he majored in Aerospace engineering and Business/economics. It's also where we met. "The only thing about living in Minneapolis is that there is so little diversity." He observes, "no one asked me when I lived in LA, 'what are you doing in LA?' Now I get this question often." To a certain degree, he's right. I learned that immigrants tend to move to populous states near centers of industry, like California, New York, or even Florida. "Why don't you move?" I asked. "It seems that you could move or work anywhere you want, with the recommendations you would get at your company." Rajat had figured out a way to save his company hundreds of thousands of dollars each year through more efficiently designed urinary catheters. For the record, I'll also add that his designs maintained industry safety standards. He was barely a year at the company before receiving messages on LinkedIn from other high ranking companies in Silicon Valley. "Well, I don't wish to seem opportunistic. My boss hired me for a 2-year commitment. Better that I leave on good terms." Honorable. Rajat and I talked quite a bit, along the many lakes in Minnesota, in various museums around the city, in Stillwater (try Nelson's ice cream), and at the fireworks around Lake Calhoun. It was an enjoyable time, celebrating the country's independence. I felt I renewed sense of pride, given the popularity of *Hamilton, the Musical.* Immigrants, like Rajat truly helped to build America, and I am inspired by the recent recognition of this history.

Our earthly governments should remind us of the heavenly, established by the Holy Trinity: Isaiah 9:7: Of the greatness of his government and peace there will be no end. He will reign on David's throne and over his kingdom, establishing and upholding it with justice and righteousness from that time on and forever.

A Fine Summer in Chicago

The zeal of the LORD Almighty will accomplish this.

A Fine Summer in Chicago

Resilience

There is something to be said for the adaptable nature of the human spirit. Yet sometimes, the fundamental goal of this adaptability, or self-preservation, can be at odds with our moral imperatives—like truth and justice. After returning from Minnesota, I felt refreshed, feeling that I needed to finish an experiment, looking at Protein Y (secondary aim) levels after transfection with a small interfering RNA. Briefly, all you need to know is that siRNA reduce levels of protein production in the cell by preventing their translation from RNA. This was a routine experiment that I learned and employed over the summer. On WB, I saw no difference in levels of Protein Y. Calling on Tim, I tried to reason that, if you squinted hard enough, it seemed there was a slight decrease in protein. "I don't buy it," he concluded. He and I then looked at my protocol to assess what went wrong. It was not until 2 weeks later, after I decided to use a new transfection protocol, that I realized I had used an incorrect reagent to reconstitute the Protein Y siRNA. Price tag: $357. I'd reached a state of Derridian aporia. Because I was the only person at the time to know what I had reconstituted the siRNA in, I could either A) Not tell a soul, try and get a new siRNA by reasoning with Grace that the tube we had ordered was defective B) Tell Colin and Grace that I had made a huge error or C) Leave the lab right that second, never to show my face in town again (Trust me, all these thoughts flashed before my eyes). The first option seemed dishonest, and a little sketchy. The last, unthinkable. So I decided to opt for the second choice. What else could I do in Chicago, except be the bigger man? I let Grace know, telling her the full cost. "What to reconstitute your siRNA in…ah no one talks about these things. It's supposed to be in RNase-free water" Grace says. I was distraught. Here was a lab that was opening its resources up for me to study and learn, and I felt as if I was wasting it. I'd even offered to pay for a new siRNA construct with my personal savings. "Of course not," Grace says, "these things happen."

A Fine Summer in Chicago

The question now was whether I wanted to continue to study Protein Y, given the mishap that entangled me from elucidating its use that summer. Not wanting to repeat my mistakes, I thought hard about whether to re-order the construct. After talking to another pot-doc, Max, for his opinions, he whispered to me with his characteristic wide-eyed demeanor: "don't do it." I even asked my father, a civil engineer with no biological training. He decided that there were worse things that could have happened, and that it was better to retry the experiment. "This is research. Things happen." I found that encouraging, and decided to reorder the construct. I spoke with Colin about it, to which I received a "You get one pass for being new, but that is a lot of money." Resilience is one form of adaptation, I think. We all have to develop a capacity for the courage to give our best efforts, sticking to the plans we know are good and true. At this point, already more than half-way through the summer, I think it was a bit challenging to wonder what the purpose of these setbacks were (I won't even mention the contaminated cell situation I had about 1 week later). I let Colin know that my study of Protein Y was becoming increasingly more bleak. He echoes my father. "This is research; remember we only publish 2-3% of all experiments we perform in the lab." On the one hand, there was a sense of shame in making my mistake. On the other, I began to develop an abiding sense of trust, knowing that if I failed, I could express that failure honestly, without being rejected. I hope that future researchers take this honesty to heart. I certainly have.

A Fine Summer in Chicago

Impact

Meanwhile, I resumed my work on Compound X, assessing its adhesive, invasive, and proliferative potential. There were larger truths to be discovered here, I believed. I had noted all the literature evincing a reduced level of ovarian cancer metastasis after treatment with the compound. Yet, in spite of this resounding belief, I was not met with any successful decrease in the three assays mentioned above. So as a consequence, I decided to make my summer worthwhile, and like Colin said, continue to "steal" the knowledge around me. This meant attending our Grand Rounds sessions, in which the physicians involved in the department of Obstetrics and Gynecology gathered each Friday morning to discuss interesting cases, or to listen to lectures from those within their cohort. The list of physicians in attendance was long, and interestingly enough, there was still an incredibly intimate, humbling level of detail shared. This was especially true as physicians shared on topics such as the dangerously elevated rates of Doppler Ultrasound use for normal pregnancies, or when they shared the mistakes made by either themselves or by other physicians within the department. I found it a highly stimulating and practically useful meeting to attend. Colin also asked me to attend the departmental Tumor Board sessions. These took place each Wednesday morning. Residents went down their list of patients, presenting the cases and any unresolved clinical questions. The physicians would generally bounce the questions around with each other. I felt it helpful too, because it was evident that in gynecologic oncology there was a strong utilization of the histologic slides. We had practiced histology a ton during our first year in almost every course. Clearly, this was for a reason. We leveraged histology to understand ovarian cancer in every single case we observed. The more practice I got at reading it, the better.

With the summer coming to a close, it was evident that two things were needed: the scientific paper that we would submit to the

A Fine Summer in Chicago

administration, due August 19th, and a 7-minute presentation that I would give at the Summer Research Project Forum on August 24th. Given my lackluster results in the summer, up to mid-August, I had to simply write my paper about my lackluster results. The entire summer though, I was editing, presenting, and re-editing my presentation as I gained new methods or results. As the summer progressed, the secondary aim of my project began to fizzle, leading to a more focused project. So as the summer progressed, my presentation and presentation skills began to grow stronger.

Incremental progress was noted in my experiments as well. I'd noticed that one patient seemed to respond to the doses of Compound X I had been giving. I think these small bursts of hope edged me on. Later on in the summer, Colin had called me in to discuss things. He saw that I was still placing a huge pressure on myself to produce something of value for the summer. "I know you want to potentially publish something, but I have to tell you, it can take years. You have worked very hard this summer. I would be ok with you going off tomorrow to see your parents and coming back on Monday," he says.

I would have been too. But, Colossians 3:23-24: Whatever you do, work at it with all your heart, as working for the Lord, not for human masters, since you know that you will receive an inheritance from the Lord as a reward. It is the Lord Christ you are serving.

I explained to Colin that my 3-week vacation was coming, but that I'd still harbored the belief that I could make some semblance of an impact.

After several more experiments with Compound X, visits to a biostatistician, and assessments of mesothelial cells transfected with siRNA targeting Protein Y, I was ready to focus solely on

A Fine Summer in Chicago

increasing the dose of Compound X.

A Fine Summer in Chicago

Auspicious Endings

After weeks of error and trial, with my final paper finally uploaded as of August 20th, and with 72 hours to go before my final presentation was due, I was now in the home stretch. Harboring one last idea, I figured I'd try it out. At this point, it should be mentioned that Shawn Cummings, the medical student who had been in the lab the previous summer, had returned for several more weeks of his experiments in the hopes of finalizing his paper for submission to a scientific journal. He and I hit it off pretty well, as fellow medical students around the same age—he at 26, and I at 24. He even introduced me to Claudia, his girlfriend, with whom I had gotten along well. Shawn and I hung out outside our long hours in the lab: having all-you-can eat sushi, and sharing food or drinks at a Polish-themed party (one of our friends in the lab was Polish). We developed a friendship that extended beyond professional. It was that personal connection with Shawn that gave me the freedom to enlist his help on Sunday the 21st, asking him to help me plate fibroblasts for a 3D culture of cells while I analyzed data for an invasion assay.[4] It was a busy day.

After I had plated the mesothelial cells on top of the fibroblasts, I gave them 16 hours of treatment with Compound X at a dose one order of magnitude above what I had been previously giving. Next, I removed the treatment, washed the cells, and then plated the layer of Ovarian Cancer cells for 1 hour before decanting any non-adherent cells. The results I got that Monday were surprising, in that, it actually worked. Across all patients tested, I saw a decrease in ovarian cancer adhesion at the higher dose. I should mention that I had shown the same effect, although more pronounced, with ovarian cancer cells in simple co-culture (without fibroblasts) using the same method of treatment. Unfortunately, time did not allow me to perform invasion and proliferation assays at the higher doses before my presentation.

A Fine Summer in Chicago

Interestingly, it seemed that cells treated at the lower dose were associated with lower levels of ovarian cancer invasion, when averaged across multiple patients. At the lower dose, I'd also seen a reduction in adhesive proteins associated with secretion by mesothelial cells undergoing oxidative stress. I do not say all of this with definitive certainty. As a friend of mine put it, "If cancer was easy to cure, we would have solved it by now." That is to say, these experiments are not definitive, and must be repeated. Still, it was an exciting couple of days. Reflecting now, I suppose these were the brief glimpses of hope that physicians of all specialties see in their medical careers. Glimpses that give them the strength to continue fighting the illnesses that plague our beautiful world. With the results received on the night of Monday August 22nd, I stayed awake until 5:30am the next morning analyzing my data, putting together my presentation, trying to seal it as my best presentation to date.

A Fine Summer in Chicago

Ending

I was scheduled to present Wednesday, August 24th. With all the
support of classmates, faculty, and some folks from the lab, I gave
my presentation with all the vigor I could muster describing the
morbidity and mortality of ovarian cancer, the way it disseminates
within the peritoneal fluid, the aim of my study repurposing an
antioxidant to fight ovarian cancer, then discussing my hypothesis,
methods, and ultimately results and discussion. I was giving a
scientific talk before my faculty and peers! I enjoyed the time I
had doing it. Of course, I was a bit nervous, as we can all be in
front of a crowd. Transitioning between slides, as I had timed
them, making the necessary tonal inflections I had practiced so
many times before, I began to gain more confidence, which
showed after the question and answer session. I went over my
allotted two minute time period in order to deconstruct the barrage
of questions I received. At the finish, I stood with confidence,
knowing I had done my absolute best to make an impact on the
field of ovarian cancer research. My talk was met with praise,
called "brilliant" by Grace, and was commended by others from
my lab, as well as from the faculty and students. Having gone
through the experience, I understand now that the setbacks of
research take time to pick apart, and the pitfalls we encounter
when we give a treatment that does not work sometimes takes a
team of people to understand, often requiring a very detailed
recollection of events by the researcher. Is this not also true of the
professional life of the physician?

 In the end, research called on me to be the best version of myself:
hard-working in the long days, patient for experiments that would
take hours or days, thoughtful when other students reacted or
failed to react to a comment/suggestion in the expected manner,
sophisticated in my experimental design, all while cracking jokes
in the hustle and bustle of camaraderie. Reflecting now, it dawns
on me that the currency among the well-educated is not simply

accomplishments—it is humor. One does not simply go through a day without making light of either him or herself. It is too hard. Tim Peterson, the post-doc that I have referred to multiple times, is an easy-going guy. He's a smoker, taking a 10 minute break every hour to feed his habit. Tim works hard, not just in experiments, but also in teaching others, helping out around the lab, and making others feel comfortable and welcome by delegating responsibility. He does this, all while sharing laughs and making jokes. It's his diligence, combined with a self-described apathetic, "Honestly, I just don't care what people think", attitude that has allowed him to accumulate the trappings of a strong researcher: several awards, 30 publications at 30 years of age—2 of which were in *Nature*. Tim still looks out for me, helping me to trouble shoot my experiments, all the while helping me to think more definitively like a scientist. For that, I am very grateful to him. He wouldn't want me to give you his real name of course, because as he puts it, "I don't want people thinking I'm nice. I don't like it." Classic Tim.

A Fine Summer in Chicago

Death Leading to Life

Not winning an award for my research this summer was fine. Given the distance I had traveled from Spring until now, the friends I've made, and the project success I've had, I don't need any recognition to validate my time in the lab. In a way, I feel that by not winning, I have gained more. Would I have felt the need to share my story with you if I'd won?

In losing, I had gained a sense of resilience. I feel that in trying to learn and master the techniques I was utilizing in ovarian cancer research, that I was becoming completely lost in what I was doing. In a way, this was good too, but I think losing brought me back to reality. One scripture stands out to me. It is John 12:24-Very truly I tell you, unless a kernel of wheat falls to the ground and dies, it remains only a single seed. But if it dies, it produces many seeds. Here, Jesus is referring to his own death, a sacrifice that would ultimately empower generations of Christians to sacrifice their own lives for his sake. Yet, I can't help but also feel that I had died to the original perspective that my project would somehow be more important to the history of the universe, and would leave some lasting legacy than the daily interactions and relationships I would have with Jesus, family, or friends. This loss was humbling, and I've seen it produce other fruits in me. In a way, I felt like Abbey D'Agostino, who collided with a teammate during the women's 5K in the 2016 Rio Olympics and lost, yet still was able to say at the end of the day "Him (Jesus) First." It was this attitude that gave her the love, determination, and understanding to help her fellow teammate cross the finish line.

I have peace this summer, and it is this peace that galvanizes me to share with you the details of the growth accompanying my new life in Chicago. More importantly, it has allowed me to illustrate how the Almighty gives us situations that ultimately result in our edification. You, my reader, being old enough to read these words,

A Fine Summer in Chicago

have surely experienced disappointing circumstances at some point. I just thought I'd share with you how God has empowered me to deal with my own.

My heart is filled with love for this city.

A Fine Summer in Chicago

References

1. Mikuła-Pietrasik, Justyna, Patrycja Sosińska, Małgorzata Kucińska, Marek Murias, Konstantin Maksin, Agnieszka Malińska, Agnieszka Ziółkowska, Hanna Piotrowska, Aldona Woźniak, and Krzysztof Książek. "Peritoneal mesothelium promotes the progression of ovarian cancer cells in vitro and in a mice xenograft model in vivo." *Cancer letters* 355, no. 2 (2014): 310-315.
2. Prendergast, Franklyn G., and Kenneth G. Mann. "Chemical and physical properties of aequorin and the green fluorescent protein isolated from Aequorea forskalea." *Biochemistry* 17, no. 17 (1978): 3448-3453.
3. Cheng, George Z., Joseph Chan, Qi Wang, Weizhou Zhang, Calvin D. Sun, and Lu-Hai Wang. "Twist transcriptionally up-regulates AKT2 in breast cancer cells leading to increased migration, invasion, and resistance to paclitaxel." *Cancer research* 67, no. 5 (2007): 1979-1987.
4. Brueggmann, Doerthe, Claire Templeman, Anna Starzinski-Powitz, Nagesh P. Rao, Simon A. Gayther, and Kate Lawrenson. "Novel three-dimensional in vitro models of ovarian endometriosis." *Journal of ovarian research* 7, no. 1 (2014): 1.